Slim
and
Healthy
The Easy Way

Elaine Ouston

Morris Publishing Australia

http://morrispublishingaustralia.com

Slim
and
Healthy
The Easy Way

ISBN: 978-0-6454766-7-5

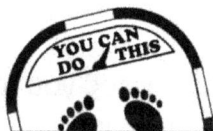

Foreword

This is not a book about using a difficult and strict diet and exercise to lose weight and keep it off. This book will give you a much easier way of doing both.

Why am I writing this book? Because I care!! It breaks my heart to watch people I love struggle with weight gain, go on constant diets, lose weight then put it back on, or worse still, risk their life and health by resorting to surgery to lose weight. I watch their health suffer because of bad choices that can be avoided.

People think I am against weight gain because of appearance. Not so! I am against weight gain because of the harm it can do to your body.

I have people say to me, "You are so lucky not putting on weight. Your metabolism must be good."

My constant weight maintenance has nothing to do with luck or my metabolism.

So, how did I maintain my weight all of my adult life and how can you lose the weight and keep it off? I'll show you how. But first I need to explain why it is so important.

If I told you that I wanted you to wear a body suit full of sand and carry that around every day, you would protest that it would be too hard, that you would get tired and that it would harm your body. What most people don't realise is that putting on enormous amounts of weight is the same as carrying all that sand.

Medical research tells me that the extra weight puts enormous strain on every muscle in your body, including the most important muscle, the heart. It also wears out the hip and knee joints. And eating more than you need also puts an enormous strain on your digestive system, as it is constantly working to digest food.

Losing weight is not an easy thing to do. I decided early in my adulthood that the most sensible thing to do was not to put it on in the first place. Many think this is not possible, but I have maintained my weight for all of my adult life, so I can testify that it *is* possible.

You can use the same method I used to maintain your weight or lose the extra weight you gained and keep it off. Going on a strict diet and heavy exercise is not needed. That way is too hard. You can do it simply by reprograming the way you think and feel about food.

Early in my working life, I attended a self-improvement course. The course taught us that the easiest way to overcome our lack of confidence to achieve our goals was to make our subconscious mind believe it was possible. They taught us that the way to do this was to write down what it is we wanted, as if it had already been achieved, clip it out and put it where we would see it every day and to read it ten times. The statement is called an affirmation and the repetition is called a mantra or a chant.

When you do this, your subconscious mind realises it is not true and works out ways to make it happen. It helped me achieve my goal of studying to become a graphic artist, even though I was working and had small children to care for. I studied at home and the affirmations kept me focused on taking the time needed to study and stopped me from allowing myself to become distracted.

At this time, I was watching the people around me putting on weight and becoming unhealthy and unable to join in the things they loved. Carrying around the extra weight was draining them of energy and making movement difficult. Even simple things like playing cricket on the beach with the kids was now not possible for some. I decided that I wasn't going to let that happen to me. So, to stay at a constant weight, I applied what I had used to achieve my career goal.

If you think that wouldn't work for you, think about this. Your subconscious mind controls everything you do. At school, we constantly programmed our subconscious mind to learn. Every morning we chanted the times tables ten times each until we could quote them without hesitation. We did the same with our spelling and everything else we needed to remember.

This is also how we learnt the rules that govern our lives, our behaviour, and our beliefs. These were programmed into our subconscious minds by our parents or teachers when we were children. It was the same with learning to drive and everything else we now do automatically.

And if you have ever tried to do something your parents taught you was wrong, you will know how hard that was. How guilt crept in as your subconscious mind kept reminding you it was wrong. That is why this method works for changing the way you think about food. If you try to eat something that your subconscious mind has been programmed to believe is a bad choice, it will bring to your mind the mantra concerning that choice and this will stop you.

Drawing on the memory in your subconscious mind is how you remember to do every single thing you have learnt.

But, before you can achieve anything, you have to be determined to make it happen and be prepared to actively work at it. Then you have to program your mind so that what you want to achieve becomes as natural as breathing.

As I said when talking about reaching my career goal, how you do that is by writing down what it is you want to remember and reading it ten times a day until it becomes set in your brain, just like your times tables and spelling.

As we go through the book, we will formulate affirmations that will reprogram your mind to help you lose weight and become healthy again, and I will explain why each one is needed. You will also find them set out in the back of the book for you to clip out and place where you believe you will see them most often.

Ideally, fix them to the fridge, the bathroom mirror, and bedroom mirror or on the window or wall over the sink. Anywhere you will stand for any length of time during the day. When you see them, consciously read them ten times. If you are standing in front of a mirror, look into your eyes as you do this, it will help embed them in your mind.

If you are worried about the rest of the family reading them, don't. If they read them and reprogram their minds, it will be to their benefit.

Programming your mind to change to this belief will take around two weeks to a month. Then, when you try to do something that goes against what you now believe, the mantra will run in your mind, and you will stop.

The mantras should be written and said in first person and present tense, as you will see.

While these statements are not true when you start using them, your subconscious mind will work to make them a reality.

So, if you are sitting on the sidelines watching other people having fun and are upset that you can't join them and want lots more energy and a healthy lifestyle, give this a go.

Let's start with the basics.

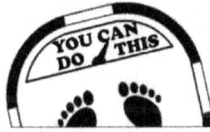

Mantra 1:

I only eat food that is good for me

Food is fuel for your body and mind. Your body can't function without it. It's just like fuelling your car. If you put the wrong fuel into it, it slows down or stops and if you flood the engine with too much fuel it tries hard to keep going but finally stops.

It's the same with your body. It needs just the right amount of high energy fuel to make it function with optimum health and strength. This comes from good food choices. Once your brain is programmed with the right food choices this will become natural and your diet will change.

When I decided to look after my body and keep my weight under control, I spent a lot of time researching and learning about healthy eating and have continued to do so ever since. I will share what I have learnt but also share information from medical authorities and weight loss services.

A vast number of foods are both healthy and tasty. By filling your plate with fruits, vegetables, quality protein sources, and other whole foods, you'll have meals that are colourful, versatile, and good for you.

People with dietary problems like food allergies or diabetes will need to adjust the foods we suggest to suit their needs.

Let's look at what the best choices are for optimum health and energy according to The Australian Government's Eat for Health Guidelines.

These are the principal recommendations featured in the Australian dietary guidelines on the www.eatforhealth.gov.au website. Check out their website to learn more.

Enjoy a wide variety of nutritious foods from these five groups every day:

1. Plenty of vegetables, including different types and colours, and legumes/beans (at least three or four different vegetables a day) and the same of fruit.

2. Grain (cereal) foods, mostly wholegrain and/or high cereal fibre varieties, such as breads, cereals, rice, pasta, noodles, polenta, couscous, oats, quinoa, and barley.

3.   Small quantities of lean meats and poultry, fish, eggs, tofu, nuts, and seeds

4.   Milk, yoghurt, cheese and/or their alternatives, mostly reduced fat. (Reduced fat milks are not suitable for children under the age of 2 years)

5.   Use predominantly polyunsaturated and monounsaturated fats such as olive oil, vegetable or nut oils, spreads, nut butters/pastes and avocado.

Good fat, especially fish oil like Omega 3, is vital for the function of your brain so make sure you get regular serves of fish, like salmon, every week.

And drink plenty of water.

Water is essential to help flush your system to get rid of toxins and to keep your kidney and heart functioning well.

Avoid intake of foods containing saturated fat, added salt, added sugars and alcohol.

1.   Avoid foods high in saturated fat, such as many biscuits, cakes, pastries, pies, processed meats like bacon and sausages, commercial

burgers, pizza, fried foods, potato chips, crisps, and other savoury snacks.

2. Replace high fat foods which contain predominantly saturated fats such as butter, cream, cooking margarine, coconut and palm oil with foods which contain predominantly polyunsaturated and monounsaturated fats such as olive oil, vegetable oils, spreads, nut butters/pastes and avocado.

3. Limit intake of foods and drinks containing added salt. Read labels to choose lower sodium options among similar foods. Do not add salt to foods in cooking or at the table.

4. Limit intake of foods and drinks containing added sugars such as confectionary, sugar-sweetened soft drinks and cordials, fruit drinks, vitamin waters, energy, and sports drinks.

5. If you choose to drink alcohol, limit intake. For women who are pregnant, planning a pregnancy or breastfeeding, not drinking alcohol is the safest option.

***

I follow these rules but because I am on a maintenance diet, I include a 'treat' of ice cream or a slice of cake once a week (or sometimes both). When I do eat treats, I limit the other foods I eat that day, so I don't take in too many extra calories.

And, although I don't make or eat cake very often, when I do make them, I use macadamia oil instead of butter or margarine and honey instead of sugar. This makes a delicious cake that is a healthy alternative.

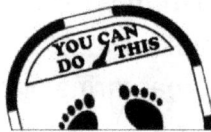

Mantra 2:

I eat 3 small, nutritious meals a day

My research tells me that there are many causes for overeating. One of them is simply that you are following the eating pattern and diet you had as a child. These eating habits have been programmed into your subconscious mind along with the rules of behaviour etc.

Another is called emotional eating. Many people crave sweet and fatty foods to gain comfort when they are feeling stressed. Depression and anxiety can also cause overeating. These cravings are a habit we need to break. Using the right affirmations will do that.

When we eat, the body uses what it needs to maintain health and give us energy to perform the tasks we are undertaking. If we take in more food than we use, the body stores it as fat to be used for energy when we need it.

But going on a strict diet by suddenly cutting out the things you have always eaten is not the way to do it. That way, your subconscious mind craves the things you stopped eating and you soon return to consuming them. Reprograming your subconscious mind is the first step.

Many people skip a meal thinking this will help with weight loss. Most weight loss service providers and the Eat for Health website will tell you that this is the worst thing you can do. One reason is that when you get hungry, as you will because your body is craving food for energy, you will snack or 'graze'. Usually this is on foods that are not the healthiest options.

Pizza, hot dogs, hamburgers, potato chips, ice cream, crisps, and other highly processed foods are loaded with trans fats. This compound clogs your arteries, raises bad cholesterol, and increases heart disease risk. It has been also linked to diabetes and stroke. Additionally, they lack nutritional value and provide nothing but empty calories that are turned to fat.

The other reason not to miss meals is that when you make a habit of going for long periods without food, your body will store what you eat in case there are more skipped meals.

Eating 3 small, healthy meals a day at regular intervals will give your body the confidence to use what you take in, knowing that more will be added when needed.

Dietitians say that it is particularly important not to skip breakfast. It has already been around 12 hours since you last ate, so you need to add food for fuel to start the day. If you don't give your body the nutrients you need, it will create hunger pains that will make you snack.

A good healthy breakfast will stop you snacking during the morning and get you through to lunch time.

Most people eat more than they need in a meal. If you follow the government food selection guidelines set out in the last section and limit your portions, you will gain optimum health and lose weight at the same time.

Once your goal weight is obtained, you can slowly increase the amount of food to a medium size meal.

By weighing yourself regularly, you can see if you are eating enough to maintain your new weight and plan meal sizes accordingly.

So, what is a Small, Nutritious Meal according to dietary experts?

For your main meal that means having a small piece (not more than 150grms) of lean meat (remove all fat) or fish or other seafood, with at least four different vegetables – a small amount of potato, a yellow vegetable (carrot or sweet potato) and two green vegetables. Eliminate all processed meats like sausages from your diet. Most contain unhealthy preservatives and a high fat content.

Now this doesn't mean you have to have a boring meal with just these things I suggested tossed on a plate for every meal. You can use your cooking skills to turn them into your favourite foods: stews, curries, stir-fries, roast dinners etc.

How they are served is up to you. Just remember to use the healthy alternatives mentioned previously if you are frying or making sauces.

Cut out eating desserts every night or have a small bowl of fresh fruit while you are trying to lose weight. Once you are on a maintenance diet, give yourself a treat of a small serve of your favourite dessert once a week.

For lunch, a sandwich with two slices of wholemeal or mixed grain bread, with meat or fish and salad or a healthy spread of your choice, or a bowl of meat and salad is all you need.

<u>Avoid all fried foods for breakfast</u>. As the food guide says, bacon is not a healthy meat choice. Eliminate it from your diet. Try fruit and yogurt, a healthy cereal like muesli with skim milk or yogurt, or a poached egg on toast with grilled or fresh tomato and mushrooms. If you eat cereal, look for the ones with the lowest sugar content and eat only a small serve with skim milk.

I believe in the principle of 'energy in should equal energy out'. If I am having a hard labour day in the garden, taking long walks on the beach, or exploring new territory, I will eat a <u>little</u> more food than if I am sitting at the computer all day, especially of the protein foods or carbohydrates. So, if you do a job that uses a lot of energy, add a little more protein and carbohydrates for breakfast. (An extra egg and one more slice of toast or a thick shake of banana and skimmed milk instead of a coffee). But don't go overboard.

Many mothers say they don't have time for breakfast because they are busy feeding kids and getting them ready for school. The solution is to grab a banana and eat that while you are packing lunches, feeding the kids, etc. I have done this, many times.

Any dietitian will tell you that bananas are a super food. Primarily composed of carbs, they contain decent amounts of several vitamins, minerals, and antioxidants. Potassium, vitamin C, catechin, and resistant starch are among their healthy nutrients. And best of all, they satisfy your body's craving for nutrients and are filling, so you don't get hungry.

If you feel you need more food, eat a muesli bar on the way to school drop off or work.

What do we eat in our household?

Remember, ours is a maintenance diet. If you are trying to lose weight and you don't have an active lifestyle you will need to eat less.

Breakfast is a bowl of fresh fruit salad, (usually 3 or 4 different fruits in season. It always contains banana because of the enormous health benefits). We add a couple of dessert spoons of mixed nuts and cranberries on top, a couple of spoons of yoghurt on top of that, and a sprinkle of muesli.

It is a delicious and healthy meal and keeps away the hunger pains for 4 or 5 hours. Because it contains fruit sugars, protein, and starches it gives all the energy we need to get through the morning.

Many people say that cutting up the fruit takes too much time, but it doesn't take much more time than waiting for toast to cook and topping it with spread. And a whole lot less time than cooking eggs, etc. If we are travelling and can't have this, we have scrambled or poached eggs on toast.

Lunch is two slices of bread or two rice thins with either chicken, fish, cheese, or egg and a couple of salad vegetables, like tomato and lettuce, or spreads like jam and peanut paste. We use avocado as our main spread. This adds a delicious taste, is low fat and a healthy alterative to butter or margarine.

Dinner is varied, but each small serve always contains lean meat or fish (salmon is a favourite) and lots of fresh vegetables steamed, mashed, or stir-fried. These ingredients are used to make many delicious meals from curries and stir-fries to baked meals. We add fresh herbs and spices for flavour.

We only eat dessert once a week. That is usually a small bowl of ice cream with fruit and a sprinkle of grated dark chocolate on top. (Lindt 70% coco butter chocolate with no animal fat is a favourite).

Sometimes when we are out, we will have a slice of cake with a coffee for lunch as a treat. But when we do, we don't eat again until dinner, so we don't add extra calories to our usual diet. We don't do this every day, just once a week.

This is not a good idea if you are trying to lose weight, but as our diet is a maintenance one, and yours will be once you reach your goal weight, this will do no harm as long as it is not extra calories for the day.

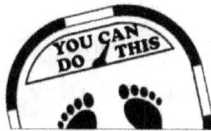

Mantra 3:

Between meals I only eat small quantities of fruit or vegetables

Snacking or grazing between meals is the worst thing you can do. Your body is so busy processing food it has no time to repair damaged cells to maintain optimum health. It needs a break between meals to do this. It also means that it has to keep storing the food away as fat, which also takes time and energy.

If you have eaten a good nutritious meal, there is no need to eat between meals and it will only be habit making you do it. Using this mantra will get rid of that habit.

I rarely eat between meals but if I do, it will be an apple, or some dried apricots, or a slice of watermelon.

People ask me if I ever eat sweets. Yes, of course. I love chocolate but I only allow myself to have one square of a dark, pure cocoa butter chocolate once a week. The one with no animal fat.

Yes, it takes discipline not to eat more but my mantra on sweets said, "I only eat one square of chocolate once a week." So, if I try to eat more, the mantra plays in my head, and I stop.

If I love it so much, why did I limit myself from eating more? Because it contains fat and sugar, and both put on weight and are unhealthy.

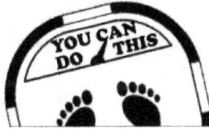

Mantra 4

I only eat a small serve of dessert and sweet treats once a week

Remember the recommendation from the Australian Government's Eat for Health Guidelines: Avoid foods high in saturated fat, such as many biscuits, cakes, pastries, and those containing added sugars such as confectionary.

If you are in the habit of eating desserts like cake, ice cream, custards, or sweets, like chocolate or lollies every day, use this mantra to help you limit the intake of the fats and sugars in these foods.

The day and time you eat them can vary but try to stick to the same day if you can.

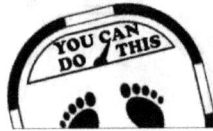

Mantra 5:

I only drink water, fruit juice and other healthy drinks

Remember the recommendation from the Australian Government's Eat for Health Guidelines: Limit intake of foods and drinks containing added sugars such as confectionary, sugar-sweetened soft drinks and cordials, fruit drinks, vitamin waters, energy, and sports drinks. If you choose to drink alcohol, limit intake. For women who are pregnant, planning a pregnancy or breastfeeding, not drinking alcohol is the safest option.

Soft drink and cordial contain lots of sugar and artificial colours and flavours and should be eliminated while you are dieting and limited on your maintenance diet. Drink pure fruit juice or water instead of these sweet drinks.

Alcohol also contains many calories and should be limited or eliminated while trying to lose weight and limited on your maintenance diet.

Tea and coffee don't contain high calories on their own but if you are in the habit of adding a couple of teaspoons of sugar and full fat milk you need to limit them to one a day. Try using honey as your sweetener. It is better for you, and you don't need as much to get the sweetness you want.

If you don't want to give up the drinks mentioned, limit them to one a day.

Water is necessary to cleanse your body and help with weight loss. Try to drink 4 or 5 glasses a day.

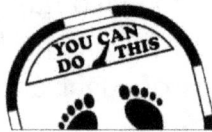

Mantra 6:

I weigh …. kgs and easily maintain that weight.

Find out what your ideal weight or your BMI (body mass index) is, using your height, age, and present weight to calculate it. There are many websites where you can do this. Or if you already know what weight you want to be, add that to the mantra in the back of the book when you cut it out.

When I was 25, my gym manager worked out that from my age and height I should weigh between 58 and 64 kg. Over the years, even after having children, my weight stayed within those guidelines. When I went to a BMI calculator online today and put in my data (height, age, and present weight) it gave me the same weight range and said, 'Continue with your healthy lifestyle."

Once you start this new plan, weigh yourself no more than once a week. Ideally at the same time of day, with no clothes to add extra weight.

Morning is best, before breakfast when your body has had time to process and eliminate the food and fluid taken in the day before. Don't be discouraged if you don't lose much at first.

It takes time for the mantra to program your mind and for your body to adjust to the changes in diet and eating habits you are making.

If you have this goal weight in your mind, when you weigh yourself and your brain registers that you are not there yet, the other mantras will become stronger.

Keep track of your loss to continue building positive habits. A Weight Loss Tracker form is at the end of the book to help you with this.

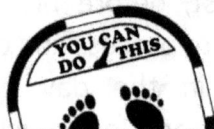

Mantra 7:

I spend at least 30 minutes, 5 days a week getting the exercise I need to help strengthen my body.

This can be a difficult one to achieve for many people – time wise and in other ways.

People with a job and a family will find it hard to fit in exercise. When I worked and had four kids at home waiting for me at the end of the day, I found it hard to get the right amount of exercise at first. But because it was important to me, I worked it out.

I used to go to the gym 3 times a week in my lunch break. I would take a change of clothes, go to the gym and exercise for 30 minutes and grab a sandwich on the way back. Or work through 30 minutes of my lunch hour, finish early and go to the gym then.

Most times, I would just hop on the walking machine for the 30 minutes but sometimes I would do a yoga or exercise class. I found that when I did this in my lunch hour, my brain functioned better in the afternoon, and I was more relaxed.

It helps if you build a support network of friends, family, or co-workers to join you. It's more fun to work out with a friend and you'll be less inclined to skip a day if you know someone is relying on your company to motivate them.

On weekends, I would go to the beach or to the park with the kids, sometimes with a neighbour and her kids in tow, and get the rest of my exercise there.

For me, because I have never had a weight problem, walking around the block, using the walking machine, or walking on the beach is easy, but if you are very overweight, health professionals say the worst thing you can do is wear out your joints walking for 30 minutes, and you must not even contemplate running.

Physiotherapist recommend using an exercise bike, doing floor exercise or yoga, swimming, or exercising in the pool, to take the stress off your joints. They also recommend that you start slowly and work up to speed over a few days to not stress your heart.

Focus on what you're capable of doing today and don't become discouraged by worrying about what you can't yet do. As your fitness improves, you'll be pleasantly surprised at the new options that come up for exercise that you will find enjoyable and challenging.

Approach your goals for health and fitness with determination and expectation. If you do this, you will succeed.

This mind programming method will help you to make positive changes to your lifestyle that will last indefinitely. It will take trial and error, as well as commitment but the result is well worth it.

Imagine the extra energy you will have when you are not carrying around all that extra weight and your health has improved.

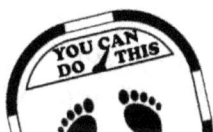

Mantra 8:

Your Mantra

Some of these mantras may not be necessary for you. Use only those that you need.

But as you progress through this journey, you may find habits we haven't covered popping up and stopping you from reaching your goal (as I did with my love of chocolate). Write a mantra that will help you break that habit. Or maybe you will need the chocolate one as well.

You can also use this method to make any other changes in your life. If you feel you lack confidence to achieve something you desire, try writing a mantra about that.

Write your own mantras to cover any other issues and paste them up with the others.

Remember to write them in first person, present tense, as if you have already achieved them, as the others are written.

Cut out the mantras that follow and put them where you will see them often. Read each one daily at least ten times.

Good luck with your journey. I hope you can achieve what I have and improve your health and lifestyle.

Remember, persistence is the key to achieving anything.

***

Disclaimer: The information in this book follows my own personal journey with weight maintenance and the results of research I have done. While I have endeavoured to provide up-to-date information from dietary experts, no claims are made as to its accuracy or validity.

This book is not supposed to replace medical advice. The author is not responsible for the actions and results of the reader. Please seek out the advice of a doctor if you are unsure if this is the right method for you. The author is not a medical practitioner and the information in this book is meant only to supplement your health decisions and actions, not dictate them.

If you have food allergies, diabetes, or other diet restrictions, please adjust the foods suggested to suit your dietary needs.

This advice has helped others lose weight and maintain their goal weight.

About the Author

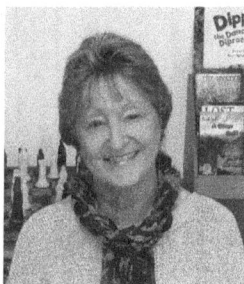

Elaine Ouston has a Master of Letters in Creative Writing and a Diploma of Graphic Art. She teaches writing to children and adults and edits for other authors.

She has many published books.

She is available for book signings and author talks about her books or her weight maintenance journey and for school talks and writing workshops.

You can find her books on the Morris Publishing Australia website.

http://www.morrispublishingaustralia.com/elaine-ouston---author.html.

And buy signed copies of her books, including this one, from her website: www.elainejouston.com.

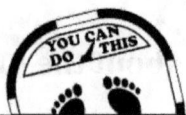

Mantra 1:
I only eat food
that is good for me

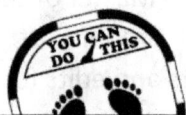

Mantra 2:
I eat 3 small,
nutritious meals a day

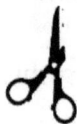

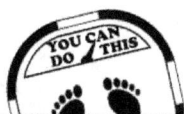

Mantra 3:
Between meals I only eat small quantities of fruit or vegetables

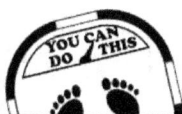

Mantra 4:
I only eat a small serve of dessert and sweet treats once a week

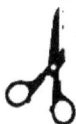

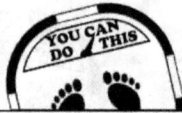

Mantra 5:
I only drink water, fruit juice and other healthy drinks

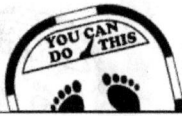

Mantra 6:
I weigh .... kgs and easily maintain that weight

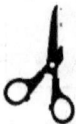

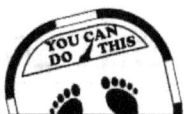

Mantra 7:

I spend at least 30 minutes, 5 days a week getting the exercise I need to help strengthen my body.

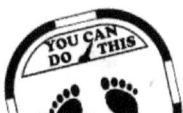

Mantra 8:

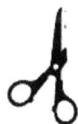

WEIGHT LOSS TRACKER

MONTH: **YEAR:**

DATE	WEIGHT	GAIN	LOSS	NOTES

www.ingramcontent.com/pod-product-compliance
Lightning Source LLC
Chambersburg PA
CBHW060703280326
41933CB00012B/2290